If cancer can, you too can, fight.

--

Vikrmn

ISBN: 9798360511397
Publisher: Elephanta Books
First Edition: 2022

DEDICATED TO...

My father
Sh. C. L. Verma
who left us after stage four.

ACKNOWLEDGMENT

I am thankful to and inspired from my Aunt
Smt. Kiran Bala to pen these thoughts down for the
courage she had shown even after the removal of
90% of her stomach due to cancer; that too with all
smiles, that's beyond imagination; setting an
example for others.

1.
Strong;
Will...

~

Strong will is a pill that will kill cancer. Cancer is a drill uphill but still, take a chill, get the courage-like skill, let it spill, let your heart fill with this little thrill and march till you grill every cancer cell to nil.

--

If cancer can,
you too can,
fight.

2.
Can;
Win...

~

CANcer

CAN't,

you

CAN,

win.

--

If cancer can,
you too can,
fight.

3.
Be that;
Story...

~

Be that story the world wants to hear; go inspire. Everyone needs motivation, not just cancer-impacted people. Be their superstar they can refer to in difficult times. Tell them how courageous you are to face cancer.

--

If cancer can,
you too can,
fight.

4.
Soul;
vs Body...

~

You are not a body but a soul; cancer can touch your body, not soul.

--

5.
Story;
vs Product...

~

Cancer is not a disease but a commodity. Don't be a product of it, be a story.

--

6.
Positivity;
To kill...

~

Negativity captured in a cell is cancer; to win cancer you have to kill every bit of negativity with positive thoughts.

--

If cancer can,
you too can,
fight.

7.
Fighter;
Not a patient...

~

Do YOU want to be known as a cancer patient, or a cancer fighter? You got it. You know it. You can do it.

--

If cancer can,
you too can,
fight.

8.
Will;
Power...

~

*Will power
will power up
your spirit
to combat cancer.*

--

If cancer can,
you too can,
fight.

9.
For;
Them...

~

Fight cancer not just for yourself but for them also who love you and want you to be with them.

--

If cancer can,
you too can,
fight.

10.
Journey;
Life...

~

The cancer journey is not easy, not simple life is either. Be strong and you will win.

--

If cancer can,
you too can,
fight.

11.
Positive;
Stronger...

~

Cancer grows faster in negativity. Be positive and come out stronger.

--

If cancer can,
you too can,
fight.

12.
Fear;
vs Courage...

~

Cancel cancer fear;
cultivate the courage
to fight.

--

If cancer can,
you too can,
fight.

13.
Soul;
Dancer...

~

*Cancer can't stop
a soul-dancer.
Be strong,
be the one.*

--

14.
Answer;
Courage...

~

Cancer isn't the answer; courage is.

--

If cancer can,
you too can,
fight.

15.
Can;
Will...

~

You CAN survive cancer because the word cancer itself has that word CAN. Build up the willpower to believe that you CAN.

--

If cancer can,
you too can,
fight.

16.
A little;
Stronger...

~

If cancer is strong,
be a little stronger
than that,
by just
1%.

--

If cancer can,
you too can,
fight.

17.
Fear;
Than...

~

*Fear of cancer
is more dangerous
than cancer itself.
Kill the fear,
before you
kill cancer.*

--

If cancer can,
you too can,
fight.

18.
Courage;
Up...

~

Courage is bigger than cancer; metaphorically and literally. Keep that courage up.

--

If cancer can,
you too can,
fight.

19.
Stay;
Go...

~

*Always tell yourself,
"I am going to stay;
cancer is going to go."*

--

If cancer can,
you too can,
fight.

20.
Who;
Created...

~

God didn't create cancer,
God created cells.
Like God created humans,
but few humans
become evil,
similarly few cells
become evil.

--

21.
Can;
Fight...

~

If cancer can,

you too can,

fight.

--

Vikrmn:

~~~

If cancer can,
you too can,
fight.

24
~~~

About

It's not just cancer that breaks people, physically and mentally, but the fear of cancer as well. It not only affects the impacted persons but other people too whom they are connected to. At that point, all need the motivation to be strong to endure tough times.

The book " **If cancer can, you too can, fight.**" injects doses of positivity to not just the cancer fighters but their family and friends too to inculcate the good vibes sparking hopes.

Vikrmn: is the author of You by You, 10 Golden Steps of Life, Guru with Guitar, 10 Alone and other motivational novels. Climate Flip, Agile Able, LIBOR Plan B and MICS Unleashed are a few of his books for professionals. The author is reachable at www.vikrmn.com.

www.ingramcontent.com/pod-product-compliance
Lightning Source LLC
Chambersburg PA
CBHW031436250726
48656CB00002B/1016